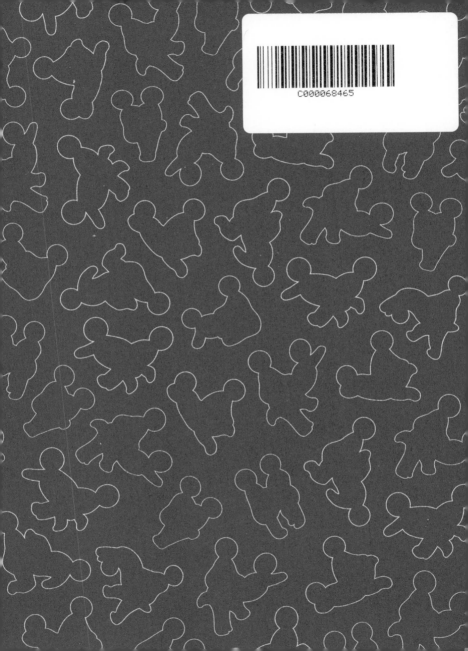

PATTI PAIGE OF @BAKEDIDEAS

THE
GINGERBREAD
KAMA SUTRA

---

25 MIND-BLOWING BAKES

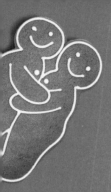
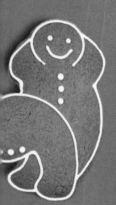
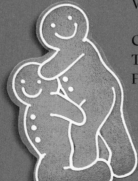

CONTENTS

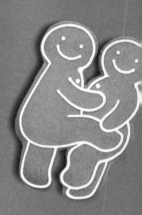

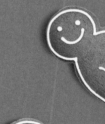
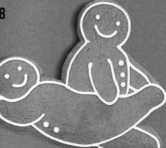

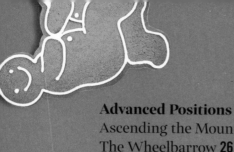

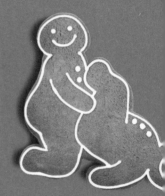

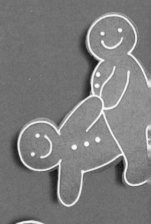

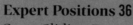

RECIPES

Patti's Classic Gingerbread

In a medium bowl, whisk together the flour, bicarbonate of soda and baking powder and set aside.

In the bowl of a stand mixer fitted with the paddle attachment, combine the butter, brown sugar, spices and salt and mix on medium speed until the ingredients are thoroughly incorporated, about 1 minute. Reduce the speed to low, add the egg and mix for another minute, then increase the speed to medium and mix for 5 seconds. Be careful not to overbeat. Pour in the black treacle and mix for 30 seconds, then reduce the speed to low.

Gradually add the flour mixture, scraping down the sides of the bowl as needed, and mixing constantly until the dry ingredients are just incorporated.

Once you have a smooth dough, remove it from the mixer and follow the instructions on pages 7–8 for preparing your dough for cutting, creating your chosen templates and cutting out your gingerbread shapes. Meanwhile, preheat the oven to 180°C/350°F/gas mark 4.

Place your Kama Sutra cookies on a lined baking tray and bake for 9–12 minutes or until slightly firm to the touch. Let the cookies rest on the tray for 5 minutes, then use a spatula to transfer them to a cooling rack. Leave to cool completely before decorating.

Makes about 30 cookies

455g (3 cups plus 2 tbsp) plain flour

1 tsp bicarbonate of soda

½ tsp baking powder

150g (⅔ cup) unsalted butter, softened

100g (½ packed cup) light soft brown sugar

1 tbsp ground ginger

1½ tsp ground cinnamon

¼ tsp ground cloves

1½ tsp sea salt

1 large egg

245g (¾ cup) black treacle

TIP: IF YOU DON'T HAVE A STAND MIXER, YOU CAN USE AN ELECTRIC HAND-HELD MIXER AND FOLLOW THE SAME TIMINGS. USE A WOODEN SPOON TO MIX IN THE FLOUR.

Vegan Gingerbread

In a medium bowl, whisk together the flour, spices, bicarbonate of soda, baking powder and salt and set aside.

In the bowl of a stand mixer fitted with the paddle attachment, combine the coconut oil and sugar and beat on medium speed for 1–2 minutes or until light and creamy. Reduce the speed to low, add the black treacle and non-dairy milk and mix until well incorporated. Don't worry if the mixture starts to look curdled at this stage.

Gradually add the flour mix, scraping down the sides of the bowl as needed and mixing constantly until the dry ingredients are just incorporated.

Prepare and bake your cookies as per the instructions on the previous page.

Makes about 30 cookies

565g (4 cups plus 2 tbsp) plain flour
3 tsp ground ginger
1 tsp ground nutmeg
1 tsp ground cloves
1 tsp ground cinnamon
1 tsp bicarbonate of soda
1 tsp baking powder
1 tsp sea salt
170g (¾ cup plus 1 tbsp) coconut oil
340g (1½ cup) vegan caster sugar
165g (½ cup) black treacle
160ml (⅔ cup) non-dairy milk (such as soy, oat, almond)

TIP: WHEN YOU'RE MAKING COOKIES WITH A TEMPLATE, IT'S IMPORTANT TO WORK FAST AS THE DOUGH SOFTENS QUICKLY ONCE REMOVED FROM THE FREEZER.

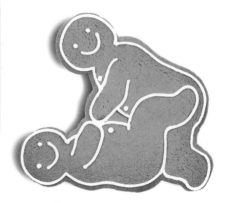

Classic Royal Icing

Makes about 240ml (1 cup) of icing

250g (2¼ cups) icing sugar

3 tbsp egg white (from about 1½ eggs), plus extra egg white or water

Sift the sugar into the bowl of a stand mixer fitted with the paddle attachment. Add the 3 tablespoons of egg white and mix on low speed for 1 minute or until smooth. Increase the speed to medium and mix for 30 seconds to 1 minute, until soft peaks just form. Scrape down the sides of the bowl and mix for a few more seconds to make sure all the sugar is incorporated. Cover the bowl with a clean, damp tea towel (this will prevent the icing from forming a crust) and set aside until needed.

When you're ready to decorate your cookies, put several heaped tablespoons of icing into a small bowl. Add drops of egg white or water, mixing after each addition until the icing is the consistency of toothpaste. The thickness of your icing is very important; if it's too thick, it will be difficult to pipe and won't adhere well to the cookie. If it's too thin, it will create a line that is too fine and difficult to control.

Decorate your cookies following the instructions on page 9.

Vegan Royal Icing

Makes about 240ml (1 cup) of icing

3½ tbsp aquafaba (the liquid from a can of chickpeas)

250g (2¼ cups) vegan icing sugar

Pour the aquafaba into the bowl of a stand mixer fitted with the paddle attachment. Beat on medium speed until it starts to foam, then sift in the sugar and beat on low speed for 30 seconds. Increase the speed to medium and beat for 3–4 minutes until soft peaks just form.

Cover the bowl with a clean, damp tea towel and set aside until needed.

TIP: IF YOUR ICING IS TOO THIN TO PIPE WITH, GRADUALLY ADD MORE ICING SUGAR UNTIL IT RETURNS TO THE RIGHT CONSISTENCY.

TIPS & TRICKS

Preparing Your Dough

Once you have made your gingerbread dough using one of the recipes on page 4 or 5, you need to let it firm up in the freezer to get the best results.

To do this, divide your dough into three pieces and place each third between two pieces of baking parchment. Working on top of the baking parchment, roll each third out until it is just less than 5mm (¼in) thick. Then stack all three slabs of dough on top of each other, place on a baking tray and put the whole lot into the freezer for at least an hour or until firm. The colder the dough is, the easier it is to cut.

When you're ready to cut out your gingerbread shapes, remove one of the pieces of dough from the freezer, peel off both pieces of parchment and cut off a piece of dough just big enough for your template. Place the piece of dough on a floured cutting board. Replace the pieces of parchment on the remainder of the slab and return it to the freezer. The dough will keep in the freezer for up to three months.

Tip: It's important to roll your cookies out to the correct thickness – if they're too thick, they will spread when they bake and lose their shape. If this happens, try rolling your cookies slightly thinner next time.

Creating Templates

Turn to the templates on pages 50–63, select your position and use a piece of tracing paper or baking parchment and a pencil to draw around the outline. Cut out your shape and draw around it once more, this time onto thicker card.

You now have a sturdy template that can be re-used to cut out several cookies.

Tip: You can laminate your templates to make them last longer and stop them picking up oils from the gingerbread dough that will cause them to bend over time.

Using Your Templates

First, prepare your work surface by dusting a cutting board with flour.

Take a piece of gingerbread dough just large enough for your template (see instructions on page 7) and place it on the board. Lightly dust the top of the dough with flour; this will keep the template from sticking.

Place your template on top of the dough. Gently hold the template in place with one hand, then cut around it using a small, sharp knife. Try to use short, small cuts to keep the dough from tearing. Leave the template in place and carefully peel the extra dough from around the edges of the cut shape. Then use your hands or a spatula to move your cookie to a baking tray lined with baking parchment. Before you remove the template, smooth out any rough edges of the dough with the tip of your knife and use a toothpick to sharpen the indents of your shape.

Now, carefully remove the template. You can still adjust the cookie at this point if you need to, but be careful not to change the shape.

Tip: If at any time during this process the dough seems too soft to work with, put the cutting board or baking tray, dough included, back into the freezer for at least 15 minutes, or until the dough has firmed up, then carry on where you left off.

Decorating Your Cookies

Once the cookies are baked and you've prepared your icing using one of the recipes on page 6, it's time to decorate!

Fit an icing bag with a #1.5 or #2 metal piping tip. Add icing to the bag, making sure you leave plenty of room to close the top completely, otherwise the icing can leak out when you squeeze. Try piping a few lines onto a piece of paper to check you're happy with the consistency, then begin to decorate your cookies. There are two ways to approach this:

1. You can look at the photos of the gingerbread Kama Sutra cookies on pages 12–49 as a guide and decorate free-hand. Don't worry if you make a mistake, you can carefully remove icing errors with a small, sharp knife.

2. If you want more of a guide, you can hold your template against the cookie and trace around it with a fine-point edible marker or the point of a straight pin. Then pipe the icing on top of the guideline to create the outline of the design, before free-hand piping the interior lines and details.

Once piped, allow the icing lines to harden for at least an hour before handling your cookies. If you're going to package them, let them harden for 6–8 hours. The buttons tend to take the longest to dry!

Tip: If you don't have an icing bag, you can use a triangle of baking parchment folded into a cone. No piping tips? Just cut a very small hole in the end of your icing bag or cone – but don't cut too much off at once, start very small and go bigger until you have the size you need.

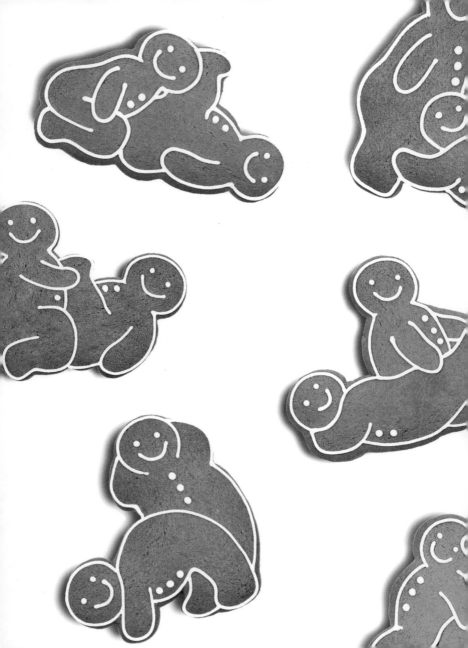

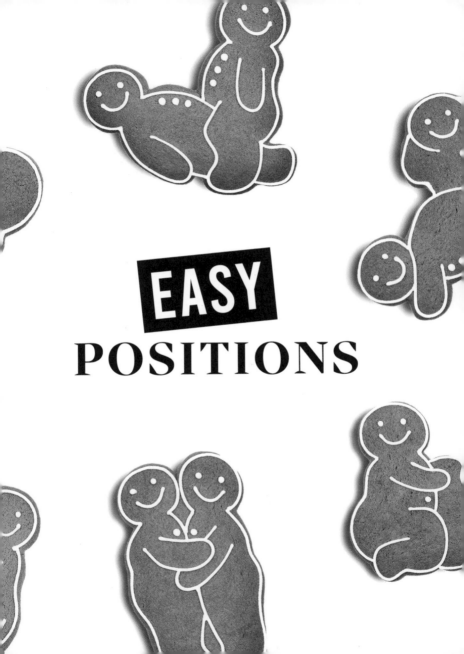

EASY
POSITIONS

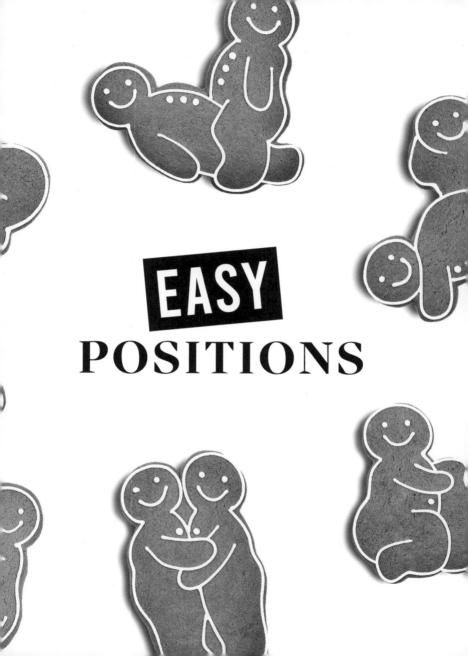

EASY
POSITIONS

EMBRACE OF THE FOREHEAD

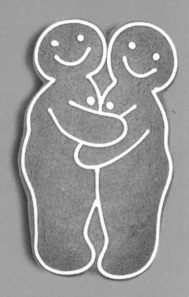

A SWEETLY LAZY LOVE-IN, THIS GENTLE EMBRACE HELPS YOU CONNECT WITH YOUR PARTNER. YOU CAN INCORPORATE IT INTO YOUR LOVE-BAKING, OR JUST USE IT AS A COZY CUDDLE. ALL YOU KNEAD IS LOVE.

Gingerbread people: Lean toward each other with your arms around one another and your foreheads touching. You should be close enough to nibble off your partner's icing smile (but resist the temptation). If gingerbread people had noses, you could rub them together.

🔥 SPICE LEVEL
More sugar than spice, consider this a dusting of powdered sugar that will boost the sweetness of any embrace.

THE SHAMPOOER

DON'T LET THE FACT THAT GINGERBREAD PEOPLE DON'T HAVE HAIR PUT YOU OFF. THIS SENSUAL HEAD MASSAGE WILL HELP YOU FEEL CLOSE TO YOUR PARTNER AND IS A PERFECT WAY TO PREHEAT YOUR OVEN.

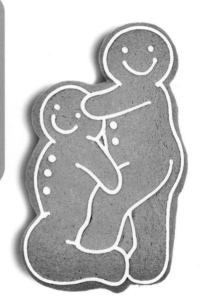

Gingerbread person one: Kneel or sit comfortably with your back to your partner. If you like, you can reach back and touch their rolling pin.

Gingerbread person two: Massage your partner's scalp. Imagine you're shampooing their hair and use gentle, soothing movements. If they like it, you can increase the pressure. (But not too much, you don't want their head to snap off in your hands. That's a total mood-killer.)

🔥 **SPICE LEVEL**
Mild but magical.

EMBRACE OF THE CALF

> IF YOUR LEG MUSCLES ARE FEELING A LITTLE CRUNCHY AFTER TOO LONG IN THE OVEN, THIS GENTLE MASSAGE COULD BE JUST WHAT YOU KNEAD.

Gingerbread person one: Lie comfortably on your front with your head resting on your arms. Let your partner lift up whichever one of your legs they're going to massage first.

Gingerbread person two: Sit alongside your partner, facing toward their feet. Gently lift up their leg and smooth your thumb along the length of their calf muscle. Repeat until the tension is gone: their dough should feel smooth and firm.

🔥 SPICE LEVEL
This might seem pretty vanilla, but it's a sweet and sensual moment with the one you love, and a great way to get things heating up between the cookie sheets.

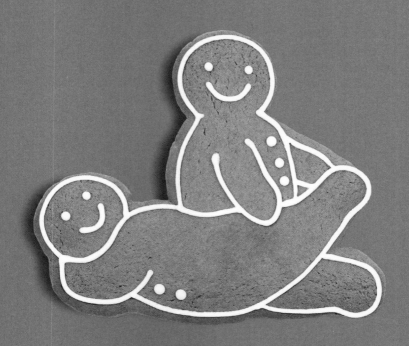

ZEUS

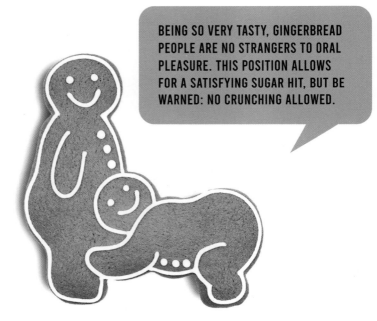

BEING SO VERY TASTY, GINGERBREAD PEOPLE ARE NO STRANGERS TO ORAL PLEASURE. THIS POSITION ALLOWS FOR A SATISFYING SUGAR HIT, BUT BE WARNED: NO CRUNCHING ALLOWED.

Gingerbread person one: Stand facing your partner, with your legs shoulder-width apart. Prepare for pleasure.

Gingerbread person two: Kneel in front of your partner's sugary bits and go to town. You can increase the spice level of this position by gently fondling your partner's nutmegs, or even reaching around to caress their buttocks – although the latter is easier for human couples, who tend to have longer arms than gingerbread people.

🔥 SPICE LEVEL
Adds a touch of cinnamon to proceedings.

WORSHIPPING AT THE JEWEL TERRACE

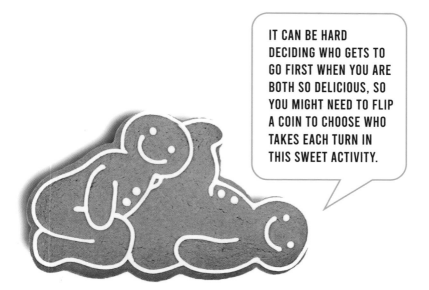

IT CAN BE HARD DECIDING WHO GETS TO GO FIRST WHEN YOU ARE BOTH SO DELICIOUS, SO YOU MIGHT NEED TO FLIP A COIN TO CHOOSE WHO TAKES EACH TURN IN THIS SWEET ACTIVITY.

Gingerbread person one: Lie comfortably on your back with your legs apart (or even up in the air, if you like). Make sure your partner has easy access to your most delicious bits. Keep that icing smile big and enjoy what's coming.

Gingerbread person two: Kneel between your partner's legs and enjoy the sweetness. Resist the urge to nibble, though, or you might not get your own turn.

🔥 **SPICE LEVEL**
Things are heating up – there's a definite ginger hit here.

CONGRESS OF THE COW

> YOU MIGHT BE MORE FAMILIAR WITH THIS AS A VARIATION ON DOGGY STYLE. IT'S A FUN AND FRISKY POSITION WITH PLENTY OF ROOM FOR MANOEUVRE.

Gingerbread person one: Bend over so you're on your hands and feet. Get that gingerbread butt up in the air and flash your partner an inviting icing smile.

Gingerbread person two: Enter your partner from behind – you might need to bend your knees a little to get the right angle. You can freestyle with your hands: hold on to your partner's hips, caress their cinnamon buns, or just rest your hands on your head like a total gingerbread G. Just baking care of business.

🔥 SPICE LEVEL
This position allows for real depth (of flavour).
Have a glass of milk on hand.

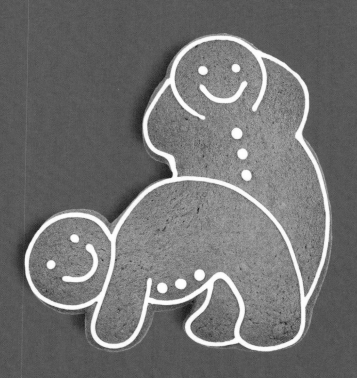

THE MARE

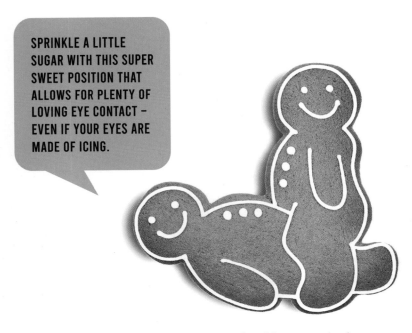

SPRINKLE A LITTLE SUGAR WITH THIS SUPER SWEET POSITION THAT ALLOWS FOR PLENTY OF LOVING EYE CONTACT – EVEN IF YOUR EYES ARE MADE OF ICING.

Gingerbread person one: Lie comfortably on your back with a satisfied smile.

Gingerbread person two: Straddle your partner, facing them, and enjoy the ride. You're in control here, so invite your partner to caress your jelly beans or play with your sprinkles. All good things must crumb to an end, so work together for a satisfying finish.

🔥 SPICE LEVEL
Perfect for a sweet tooth.

FIXING A NAIL

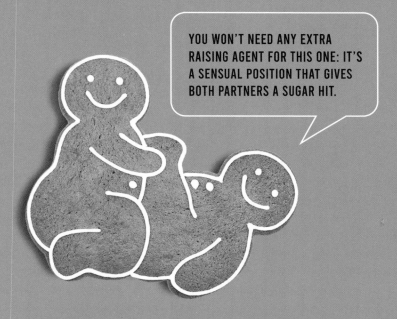

YOU WON'T NEED ANY EXTRA RAISING AGENT FOR THIS ONE: IT'S A SENSUAL POSITION THAT GIVES BOTH PARTNERS A SUGAR HIT.

Gingerbread person one: Come into a low kneeling position with your butt resting on your heels. Face your partner, ready to rock and roll.

Gingerbread person two: Lie on your back and rest your feet on your partner's chest. Lift up your gingerbread butt and wriggle yourself into position. Move together to establish a tasty rhythm.

🔥 **SPICE LEVEL**
Warm notes of cinnamon with a fiery finish.

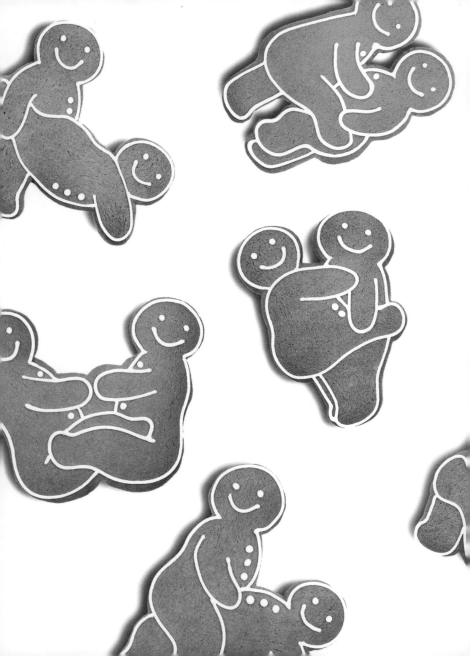

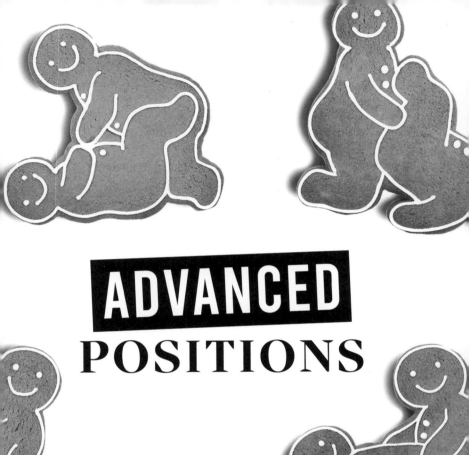

ADVANCED
POSITIONS

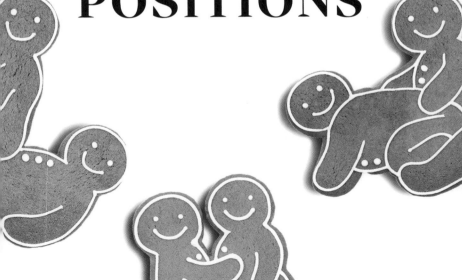

ASCENDING
THE MOUNTAIN

> A CLASSIC STANDING POSITION
> THAT REQUIRES REAL UPPER
> BODY STRENGTH, THIS ONE IS
> FOR TOUGH COOKIES ONLY.

Gingerbread person one: Stand facing your partner, with your legs slightly bent and feet apart so you'll be able to keep your balance. Brace yourself.

Gingerbread person two: Climb aboard! Wrap your legs around your partner's hips and hold on tight to their shoulders. Your partner will need to support your weight, so make sure their arms are sturdy (as all gingerbread limbs should be). You'll be face to face, so enjoy some icing-sweet kisses, too.

🔥 SPICE LEVEL
You're sure to work up a sweet, I mean, sweat.

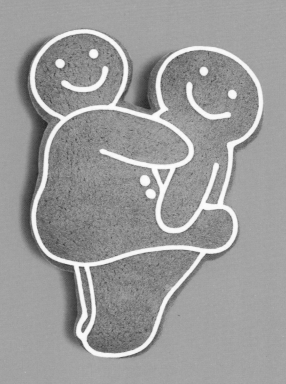

THE WHEELBARROW

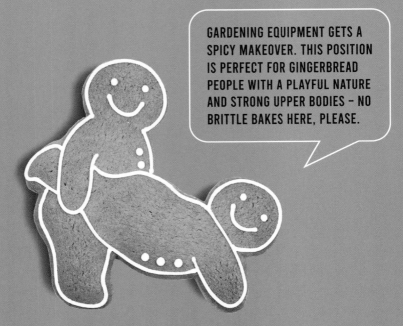

GARDENING EQUIPMENT GETS A SPICY MAKEOVER. THIS POSITION IS PERFECT FOR GINGERBREAD PEOPLE WITH A PLAYFUL NATURE AND STRONG UPPER BODIES – NO BRITTLE BAKES HERE, PLEASE.

Gingerbread person one: Bend forward on to your hands with your back to your partner, ready to be lifted into position.

Gingerbread person two: Stand behind your partner with your feet firmly planted shoulder-width apart. When you're both ready, lift up your partner's legs until you're in a wheelbarrow position and enter them from behind. Hold on tight – this is not a time for dunking.

🔥 **SPICE LEVEL**
Phew! Someone pass the chilli flakes.

RABBIT ON THE GROUND

WE'VE ALL HEARD THE PHRASE 'AT IT LIKE RABBITS', RIGHT? WELL, ONCE THE BUNNIES SEE YOU WORKING THIS POSITION, THEY'LL START SAYING 'AT IT LIKE GINGERBREAD PEOPLE'.

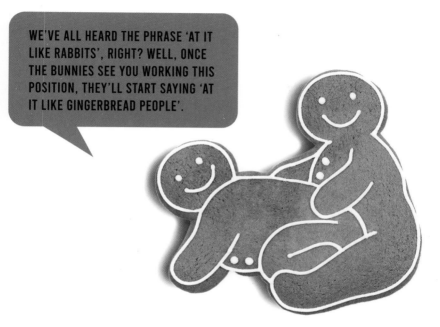

Gingerbread person one: Get on your hands and knees. Lean forward so your chest is close to the ground and open your legs wide, keeping your knees bent.

Gingerbread person two: Sit behind your partner with your legs wide open. Wriggle forward and guide your partner backward until you're in the right position. Get to it – show those rabbits how it's done.

🔥 **SPICE LEVEL**
Spice, spice, baby.

WIFE OF INDRA

ONE FOR THE MORE ATHLETIC AMONG YOU, THIS WILL WORK YOUR ARMS, LEGS AND CORE – SO YOU'VE EARNED A TRIP TO THE COOKIE JAR AFTERWARD.

Gingerbread person one: Come into a high kneeling position facing your partner. Be ready to support their legs.

Gingerbread person two: Position yourself in a half shoulder stand, with your feet resting on your partner's chest and your butt lifted up, granting them easy entry. Warning: If gingerbread people had hair, yours would be about to get pretty messed up, as this is a classic "sex hair" position. Still, that's just a whisk you'll have to take.

🔥 SPICE LEVEL
It could have a bit of a kick (especially if you accidentally boot your partner in the face).

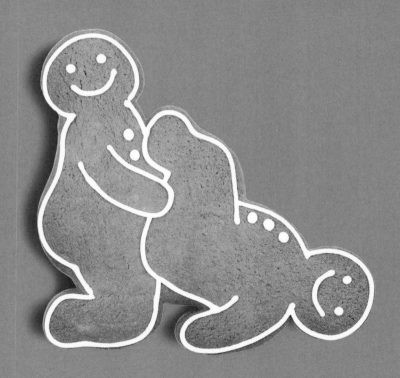

THE RICKSHAW

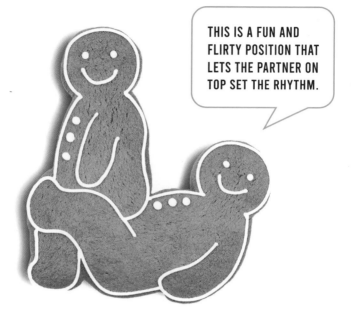

THIS IS A FUN AND FLIRTY POSITION THAT LETS THE PARTNER ON TOP SET THE RHYTHM.

Gingerbread person one: Lie on your back and raise your legs in the air. Think spicy thoughts.

Gingerbread person two: Straddle your partner with your back to them, offering them a pleasing view of your sweet butt. Rest your hands on their raised legs and begin the ride of your life.

🔥 SPICE LEVEL
Deceptive: it might seem all sugar at first, but the further you go, the spicier this ride gets.

THE PALMIST

A VARIATION ON THE MISSIONARY POSITION, THIS ENABLES YOU TO FEAST YOUR EYES ON YOUR PARTNER'S SWEET GINGERBREAD BODY AS YOU BAKE LOVE.

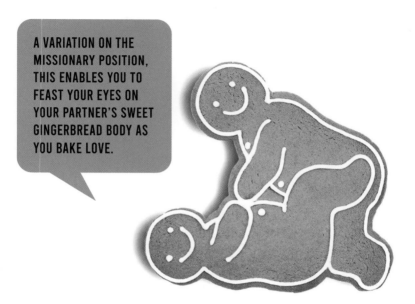

Gingerbread person one: Lie comfortably on your back with your legs apart and your arms lifted above you, palms facing up.

Gingerbread person two: Kneel between your partner's legs and lean over their body, resting your palms on theirs. Your partner can then lift their legs and rest their feet on your hips. Establish a satisfying rhythm to get things rolling.

🔥 **SPICE LEVEL**
It's getting hot in here, so take off all your cloves.

HONEY AND SUGARCANE

> THE SWEET NAME OF THIS POSITION MEANS IT IS PERFECT FOR ALL BAKED GOODS (I HEAR IT'S A BIG HIT WITH TREACLE TARTS) BUT AS ALWAYS, IT'S GINGERBREAD PEOPLE WHO REALLY BRING THE SPICE TO THIS ONE.

Gingerbread person one: Stand facing your partner. Lift up one leg and hook it over your partner's waist.

Gingerbread person two: Lift up your thigh under your partner's raised leg to help support it, then get baking. In this sexy standing position, you'll find you're up so close and personal that your buttons rub together.

🔥 SPICE LEVEL
Sugar and spice and ALL things nice.

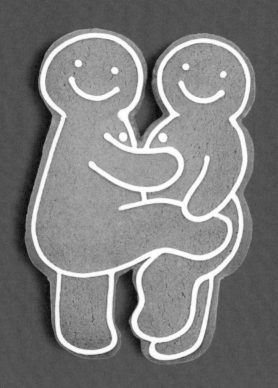

KEEN RIDER

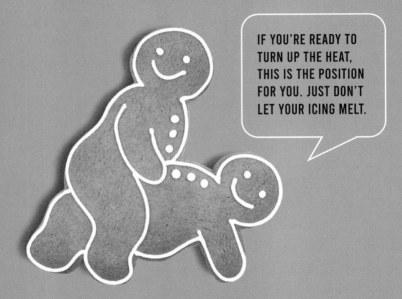

IF YOU'RE READY TO TURN UP THE HEAT, THIS IS THE POSITION FOR YOU. JUST DON'T LET YOUR ICING MELT.

Gingerbread person one: Sit on the floor. Plant your hands and feet firmly on the floor, then, with your buttons facing upward, lift up your body and hold firm. You'll need good core strength: don't crumble.

Gingerbread person two: All aboard! Straddle your partner and ride to your heart's content. Remember to keep your legs braced so you don't put all your weight on your partner. Your gingerbread thighs are gonna feel the burn.

🔥 **SPICE LEVEL**
Hot, hot, hot. You'll need an ice cream after this.

FROG FASHION

A POSITION THAT PROVIDES LOVING EYE CONTACT, SATISFYING CONNECTION AND LEAVES YOUR HANDS FREE TO EXPLORE EACH OTHER'S ICED BUNS? YOU'D BUTTER BELIEVE IT.

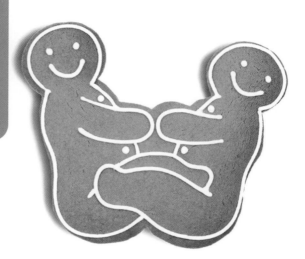

Gingerbread people: Sit facing each other with your knees bent. Wriggle as close to each other as you can and wrap your legs around one another so that one partner's legs enclose the other's body. You'll be so close together that not even a spatula could lever you apart. Move together to achieve freshly baked bliss.

🔥 SPICE LEVEL
This is a cinnamon-sweet position, with the potential to increase the heat depending on what you do with those roving hands.

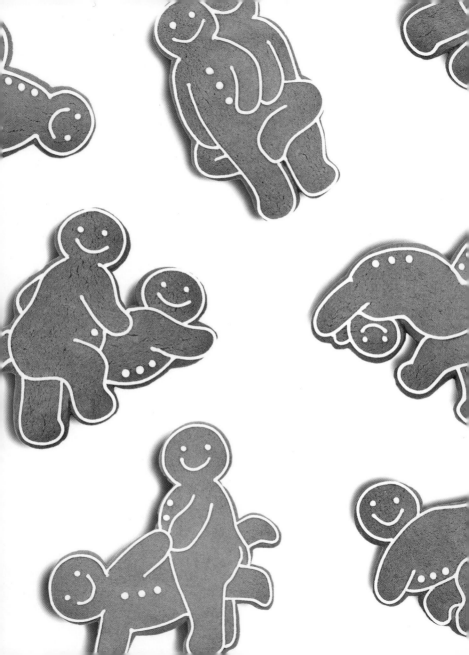

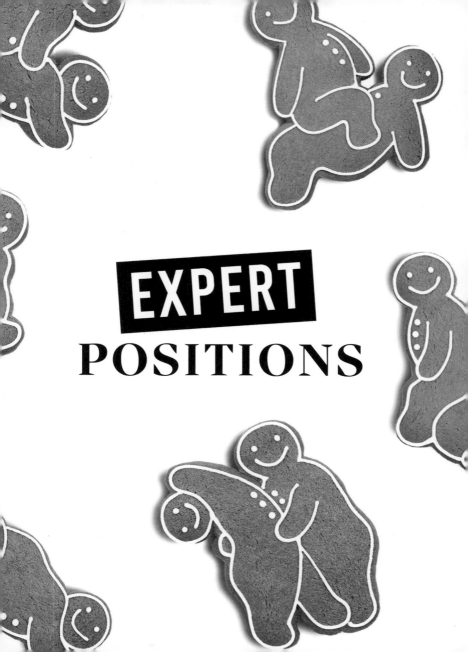

EXPERT
POSITIONS

SNOW SLIDING DOWN A HILL

A FESTIVE POSITION FOR THOSE OF YOU WHO LIKE TO CELEBRATE THE SEASON WITH SLEDGING AND SPICE. WHO CARES IF YOU END UP ON THE NAUGHTY LIST? YOU'RE GONNA LIKE IT A PUMPKIN-SPICED LATTE.

Gingerbread person one: Perform a half shoulder stand with your legs apart and picture yourself as a sexy, sensual, snow-covered... hill.

Gingerbread person two: Perch on your partner's buttocks with your knees bent. You might need to wriggle around a bit to achieve penetration, but that's part of the fun. Once you're ready, get sliding.

🔥 SPICE LEVEL
Snow or no snow, there's nothing cold about this position. It's red-hot.

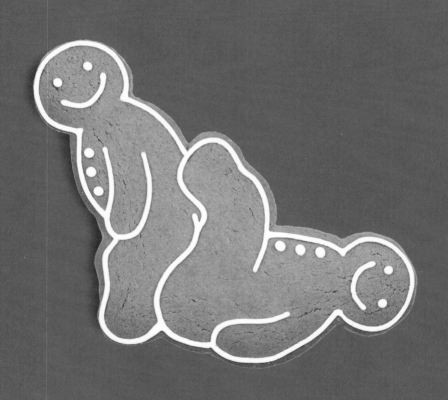

AUTUMN DOG

THIS IS CERTAINLY AN EXPERT POSITION IF YOU'RE AIMING FOR THE WHOLE COOKIE JAR, BUT EVEN IF YOUR GINGER BITS JUST DON'T BEND THAT WAY, IT'S GREAT FOR SOME SENSUAL RUBBING.

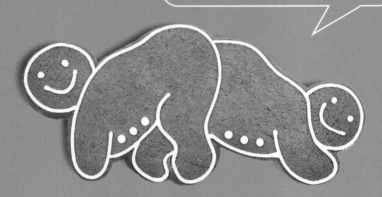

Gingerbread people: Both of you should come into a downward dog position and back up into each other until your buttocks are pressed together. Enjoy some mutual rubbing or, if you're spectacularly talented (and generously endowed in the Swiss roll department), attempt penetration.

🔥 SPICE LEVEL
For some, this will be a gentle sprinkling of cinnamon; for others, a fiery hit of ginger passion. Whatever takes your fondant fancy.

AIR RIDER

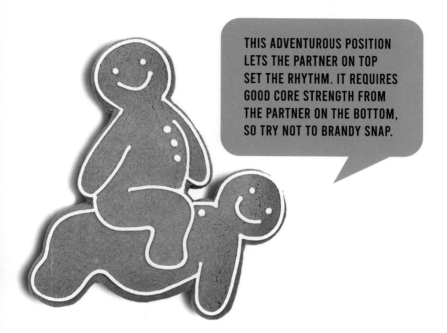

THIS ADVENTUROUS POSITION LETS THE PARTNER ON TOP SET THE RHYTHM. IT REQUIRES GOOD CORE STRENGTH FROM THE PARTNER ON THE BOTTOM, SO TRY NOT TO BRANDY SNAP.

Gingerbread person one: Sit on the floor, then lift up your body, buttons and bits facing upward, with your knees bent and your arms straight.

Gingerbread person two: Climb aboard like the scone ranger, lightly arch your back and ride, ride, ride.

🔥 SPICE LEVEL
Extra hot. You'll definitely feel the burn (in a good way).

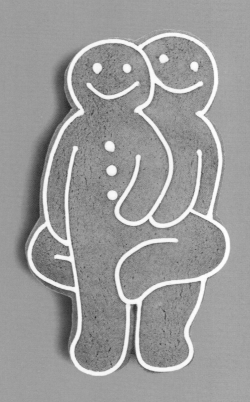

YANTRA

THIS STANDING POSITION IS ALL ABOUT SYMMETRY, BALANCE AND POISE. AND SPICE, OBVIOUSLY. UNLESS YOU ARE BOTH MASTER YOGIS, THERE IS LIKELY TO BE A CERTAIN AMOUNT OF WOBBLING, SO HAVE A MATTRESS NEARBY TO BREAK YOUR FALL OR YOU COULD BE IN FOR A FOOD AWAKENING.

Gingerbread person one: Stand on your right leg with your back to your partner. Bend your other leg so that your left foot is resting on the inside of your right thigh. Hold firm! If you're into roleplay, you can pretend to be a flamingo.

Gingerbread person two: Position yourself behind your partner so you can enter them from behind. Adopt the same position as your partner, but on the opposite side, standing on your left leg and resting your right foot against the inside of your left thigh. You can use one hand to hold on to your partner, and maybe use the other to play with their chocolate chips.

🔥 SPICE LEVEL
Have your cooling rack at the ready: this is spice-tastic.

SACRED ARCH

THIS EXPERT POSITION IS IDEAL FOR COUPLES WHERE ONE PERSON IS A LITTLE MORE BENDY THAN THE OTHER. HEY, JUST BECAUSE YOU WERE BAKED INTO A LESS EXOTIC SHAPE DOESN'T MEAN YOU CAN'T ENJOY THE SPICIER THINGS IN LIFE. CHAI THIS ONE ON FOR SIZE.

Gingerbread person one: Stand facing your partner and be ready to support them. Come into a gentle lunge position with one of your knees slightly bent.

Gingerbread person two: Stand close to your partner, facing them. When you're ready, perform a back bend until your hands are resting on the floor behind you. With your partner's help, slowly lift both legs and hook them around their waist. Your partner can ease forward until you are ready to rumble (not crumble).

🔥 SPICE LEVEL
Someone call the fire brigade: this is FLAMES.

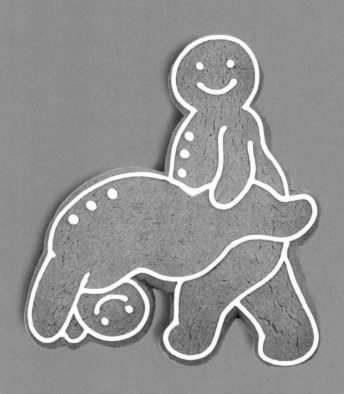

LOVE'S ARROW

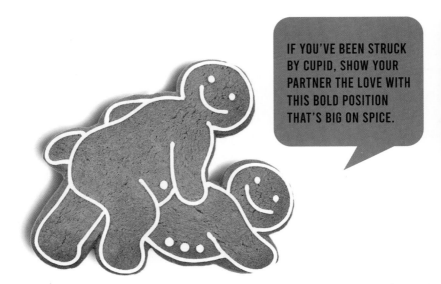

IF YOU'VE BEEN STRUCK BY CUPID, SHOW YOUR PARTNER THE LOVE WITH THIS BOLD POSITION THAT'S BIG ON SPICE.

Gingerbread person one: Bend forward on to your hands with your back to your partner. Lift one leg into the air and hold it out straight, so you're balanced on your hands and one foot.

Gingerbread person two: Enter your partner from behind, holding on to their raised leg for stability. This is a very sexy position, so try not to shoot your arrow too quickly.

🔥 **SPICE LEVEL**
Dangerously hot – you'll need to get the oven mitts out.

CRESCENT MOON

THIS IS ONE FOR ALL THE YOGA-LOVING GINGERBREAD PEOPLE OUT THERE, AS IT REQUIRES A LITTLE FLEXIBILITY. DON'T WORRY IF YOU CAN'T QUITE BEND THAT WAY – WE'RE ALL BAKED DIFFERENTLY.

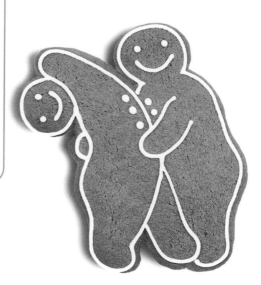

Gingerbread person one: Perform a half back bend, making sure your partner is supporting you.

Gingerbread person two: Hold on to your partner as they bend backward. Once the angle is right, you can get baking. If you're strong enough to support your partner using just one arm, use your other hand to play with their buttons.

🔥 SPICE LEVEL

A slow burn with a hint of nutmeg.

SUSPENDED SCISSORS

PHEW! THIS MIGHT JUST BE THE SPICIEST POSITION IN THE BOOK. IT REQUIRES GOOD CORE AND UPPER BODY STRENGTH, AS WELL AS EXTRA-SWEET ICING SMILES.

Gingerbread person one: Position yourself in a sideways plank position with your right hand pressed firmly into the floor, supporting your body, and your legs a little way apart.

Gingerbread person two: Stand astride your partner's right leg. Lift up your partner's left leg with your right arm and use your left arm to support your partner by holding their body or their left hand. Make sure you're both feeling steady – it's easy to lose your balance and then another one bites the crust.

🔥 SPICE LEVEL
Who knew gingerbread could be this hot?

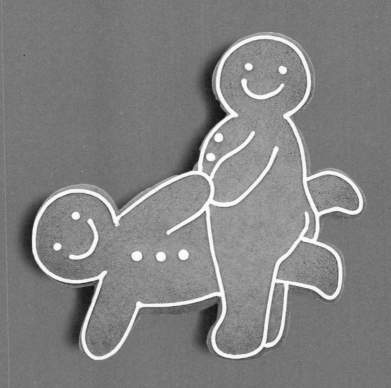

TEMPLATES

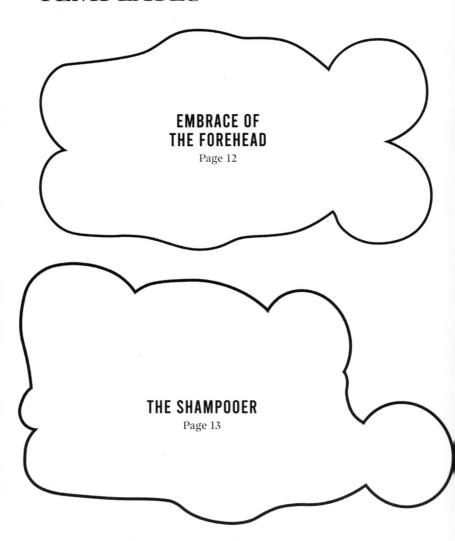

**EMBRACE OF
THE FOREHEAD**

Page 12

THE SHAMPOOER

Page 13

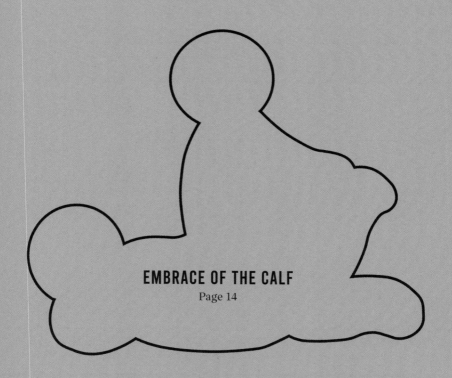

EMBRACE OF THE CALF

Page 14

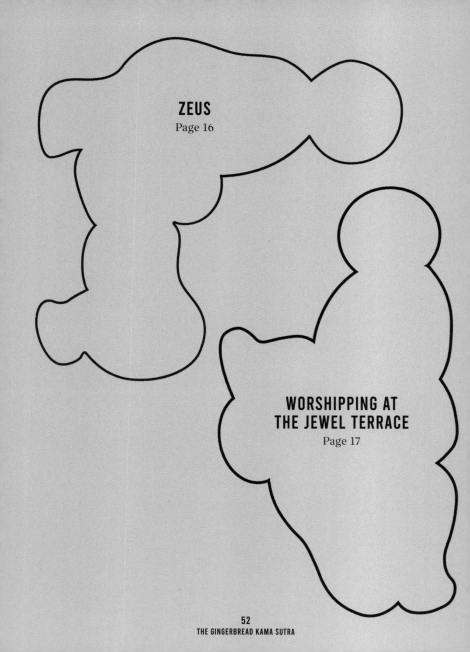

ZEUS
Page 16

**WORSHIPPING AT
THE JEWEL TERRACE**
Page 17

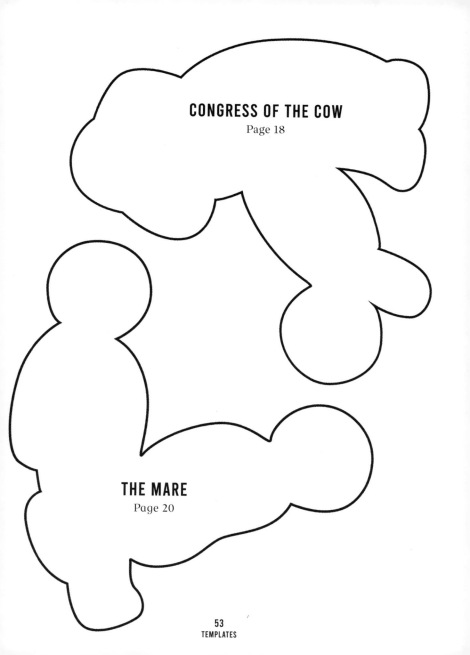

CONGRESS OF THE COW
Page 18

THE MARE
Page 20

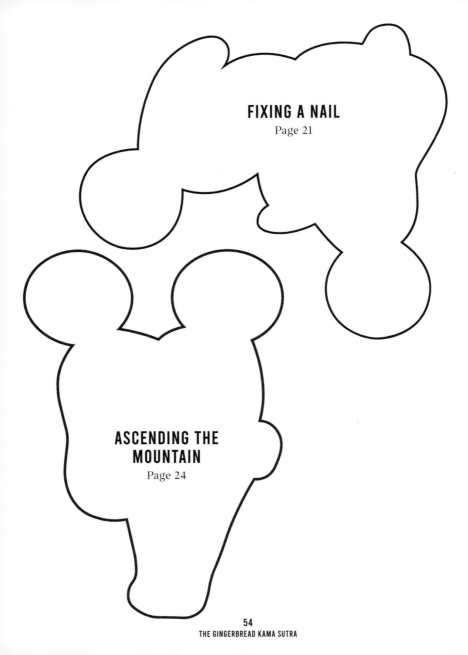

FIXING A NAIL

Page 21

**ASCENDING THE
MOUNTAIN**

Page 24

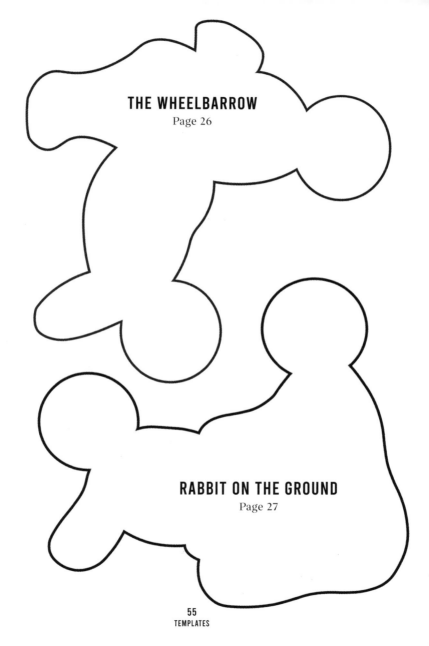

THE WHEELBARROW
Page 26

RABBIT ON THE GROUND
Page 27

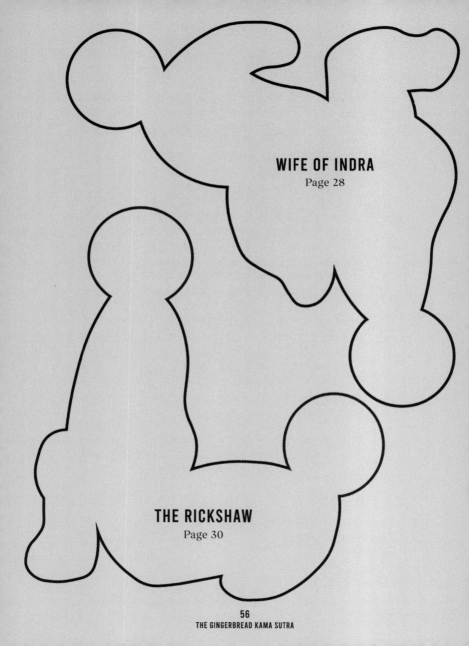

WIFE OF INDRA
Page 28

THE RICKSHAW
Page 30

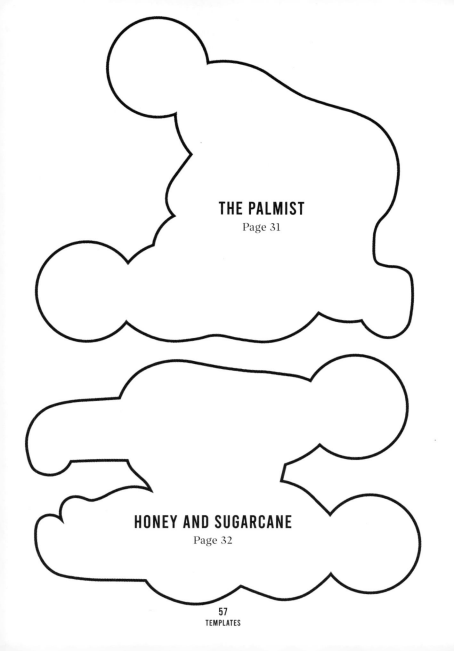

THE PALMIST
Page 31

HONEY AND SUGARCANE
Page 32

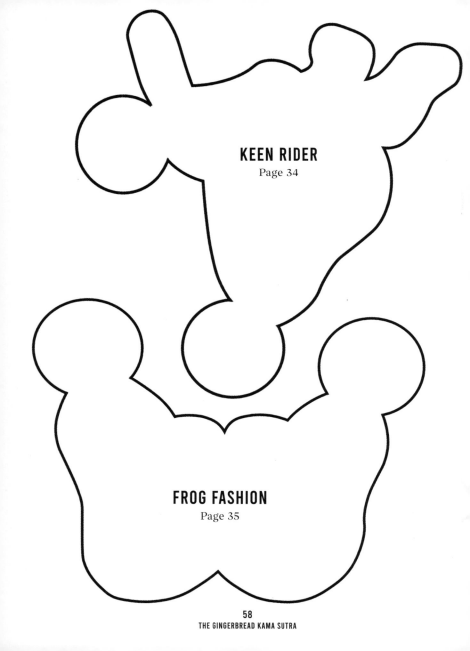

KEEN RIDER
Page 34

FROG FASHION
Page 35

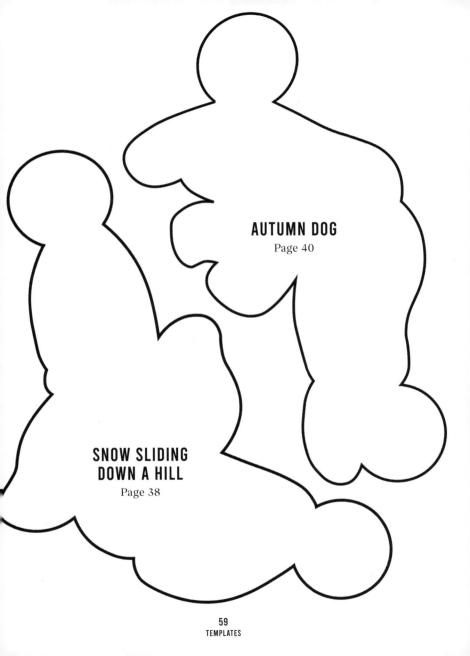

AUTUMN DOG
Page 40

SNOW SLIDING DOWN A HILL
Page 38

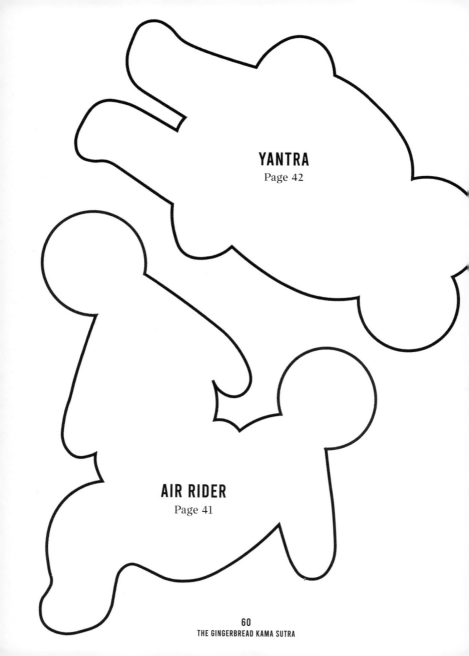

YANTRA
Page 42

AIR RIDER
Page 41

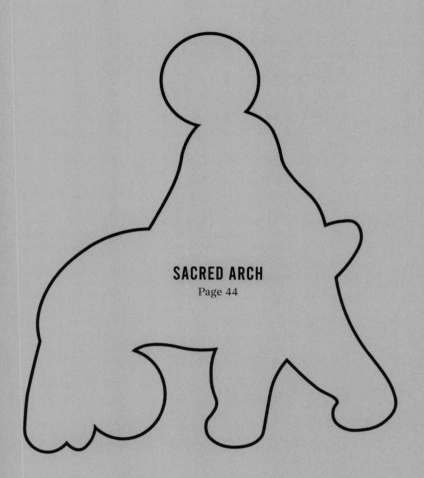

SACRED ARCH

Page 44

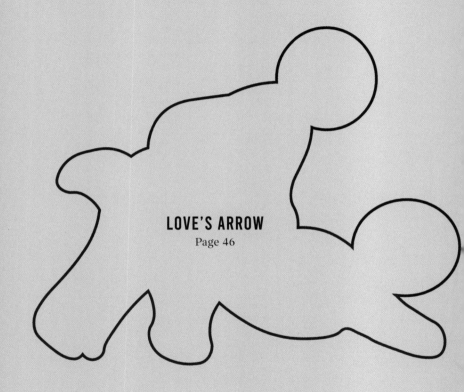

LOVE'S ARROW

Page 46

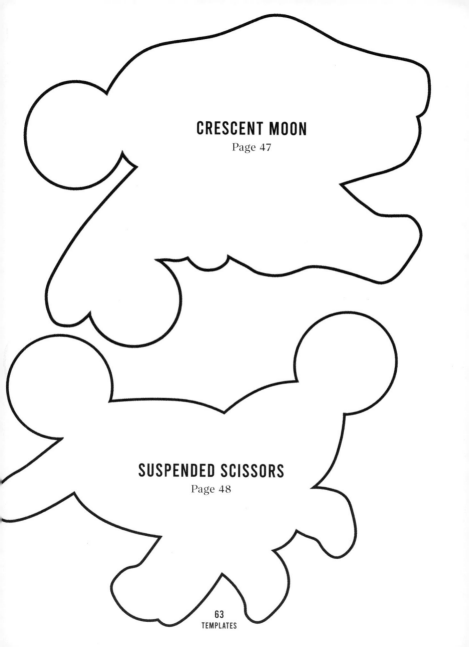

CRESCENT MOON
Page 47

SUSPENDED SCISSORS
Page 48

An Hachette UK Company
www.hachette.co.uk

First published in Great Britain in 2020
by Kyle Books, an imprint of Kyle Cathie Ltd
Carmelite House
50 Victoria Embankment
London EC4Y 0DZ
www.kylebooks.co.uk

ISBN: 9780857839213

Distributed in the US by Hachette Book Group,
1290 Avenue of the Americas, 4th and 5th
Floors, New York, NY 10104

Distributed in Canada by Canadian Manda
Group, 664 Annette St., Toronto, Ontario,
Canada M6S 2C8

Patti Paige is hereby identified as the author of
this work in accordance with Section 77 of the
Copyright, Designs and Patents Act 1988.

Publisher: Joanna Copestick
Editorial Director: Judith Hannam
Editor: Florence Filose
Design: Nikki Ellis
Kama Sutra text: Tara O'Sullivan
Photography: Goor Studio
Production: Emily Noto

A Cataloguing in Publication record for this
title is available from the British Library

Printed and bound in China

10 9 8 7 6 5 4 3 2 1

ACKNOWLEDGEMENTS

Well, what a fun project this has been! Three
flour-covered months of baking gingerbread
into every position you can imagine, and I have
some people to thank:

Florence Filose, my editor at Kyle Books, whose
excitement and enthusiasm meant I always looked
forward to our emails and phone calls. You made
the whole process stress-free and easy.

Judy Linden, my agent, for your continued guidance
and hard work, and for loving my cookies.

Nikki Ellis, for your book design that is beyond
perfect. I love it!

Tara O'Sullivan, my copywriter, for your words
that make me smile and even laugh out loud, every
time I read them.

Emily Noto, for managing the production
so smoothly.

Paul Vitale, my friend and sometimes collaborator,
for chatting about my concerns and/or technical
issues. Thanks for your always honest opinions
and good eye.

Goor Studio, for your flexibility and photography.

And special thanks to my daughter, Dena Paige
Fischer, for suggesting that I make Kama Sutra
cookies in the first place, and for creating so many
drawings for this book. You are the most talented
person I know and I love that we did this together.

UK / US GLOSSARY

baking tray – baking sheet
bicarbonate of soda – baking soda
black treacle – molasses
caster sugar – granulated sugar
icing sugar – confectioners' sugar
plain flour – all-purpose flour

Note: To measure flour or icing sugar in cups,
first use a fork to loosen it up in the bag. Then,
with a dry cup, scoop out the flour or sugar so
that it overflows the cup and sweep across the
top with the straight edge of a knife to level it off.

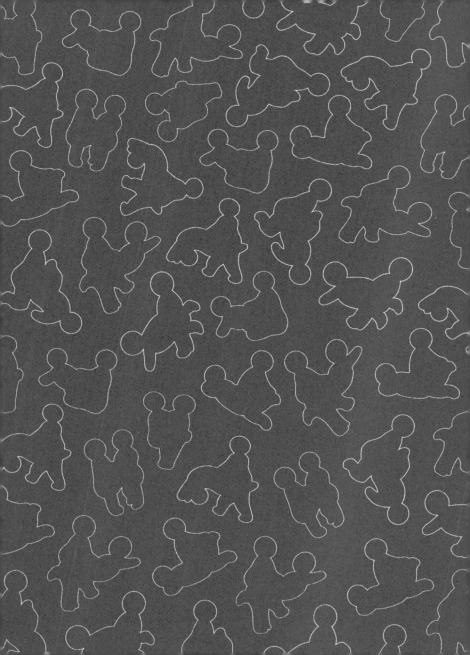